CHILDREN'S ENCYCLOPEDIA
THE WORLD OF KNOWLEDGE
ELECTRONICS AND COMMUNICATIONS

Manasvi Vohra

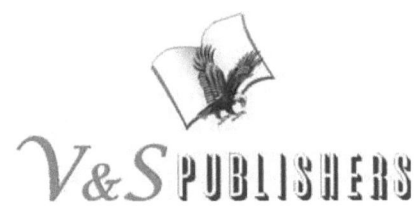

Published by:

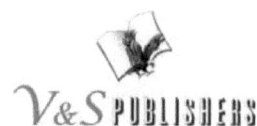

F-2/16, Ansari road, Daryaganj, New Delhi-110002
☎ 23240026, 23240027 • *Fax:* 011-23240028
Email: info@vspublishers.com • *Website:* www.vspublishers.com

Regional Office : Hyderabad
5-1-707/1, Brij Bhawan (Beside Central Bank of India Lane)
Bank Street, Koti, Hyderabad - 500 095
☎ 040-24737290
E-mail: vspublishershyd@gmail.com

Branch Office : Mumbai
Jaywant Industrial Estate, 2nd Floor-222, Tardeo Road
Opposite Sobo Central, Mumbai - 400 034
☎ 022-23510736
E-mail: vspublishersmum@gmail.com

Follow us on:

All books available at **www.vspublishers.com**

© Copyright: V&S PUBLISHERS
Edition 2017

The Copyright of this book, as well as all matter contained herein (including illustrations) rests with the Publishers. No person shall copy the name of the book, its title design, matter and illustrations in any form and in any language, totally or partially or in any distorted form. Anybody doing so shall face legal action and will be responsible for damages.

Printed at Repro Knowledgecast Limited, Thane

PUBLISHER'S NOTE

V&S Publishers is glad to announce the launch of a unique, set of 12 books under the head, *Children's Encyclopedia – The World of Knowledge.* The set of 12 books namely – *Physices, Chemistry, Space Science, General Sceince, Life Science, Human Body, Electronics & Communications, Scientists, Inventions & Discoveries, Transportation, The Earth, and GK (General Knowledge)* has been especially developed keeping in mind the students and children of all age groups, particularly from 6 to 14 years of age. Our main aim is to arouse the interest and solve the queries of the school children regarding the various and diverse topics of Science and help them master the subject thoroughly.

In the book, *Electronics and Communications,* the author has broadly dealt with some interesting topics like Introduction to Electronics, Transistor, Transformer, Capacitor, Inductor, Resistor, Introduction to Communication, Telephone, Radio, Television, The Internet, etc.

Each chapter is followed by a section called **Quick Facts** that contains a set of interesting and fascinating facts about the topics already discussed in the chapter. At the end of the book a **Glossary** of difficult words and scientific terms to make the book complete and comprehensive is given.

Quick Facts

- We can see about 2,000 stars in the sky on a clear, dark night.

Though our aim is to be flawless, but errors might have crept in inadvertently. So we request our esteemed readers to read the book thoroughly and offer valuable suggestions wherever necessary to improve and enhance the quality of the book. Hope it interests you all and serves its purpose well.

CONTENTS

Electronics and Communications

Chapter 1 : Introduction to Electronics 9

Chapter 2 : Electric Charge and Electric Current   12

Chapter 3 : Transistor   16

Chapter 4 : Transformer   19

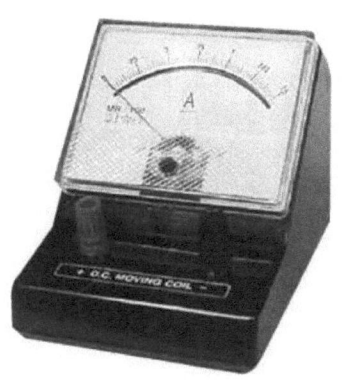

Chapter 5 : Capacitor   22

Chapter 6 : Inductor   25

Chapter 7 : Resistor   28

Chapter 8 : Uses of Electronics   31

Chapter 9 : Introduction to Communication   34

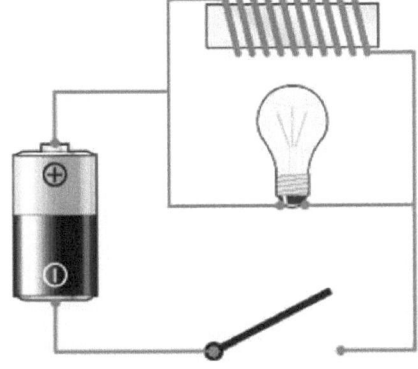

Chapter 10 : Types of Communications   37

Chapter 11 : Post and Telegraph 40

Chapter 12 : Telephone   43

Chapter 13 : Newspapers and Magazines   46

Chapter 14 : Radio 49

Chapter 15 : Television   52

Chapter 16 : The Internet 55

Glossary   58

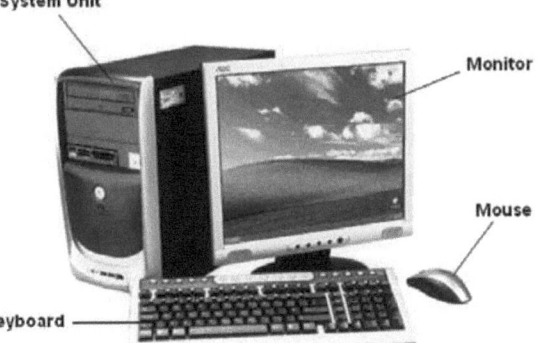

ELECTRONICS & COMMUNICATIONS

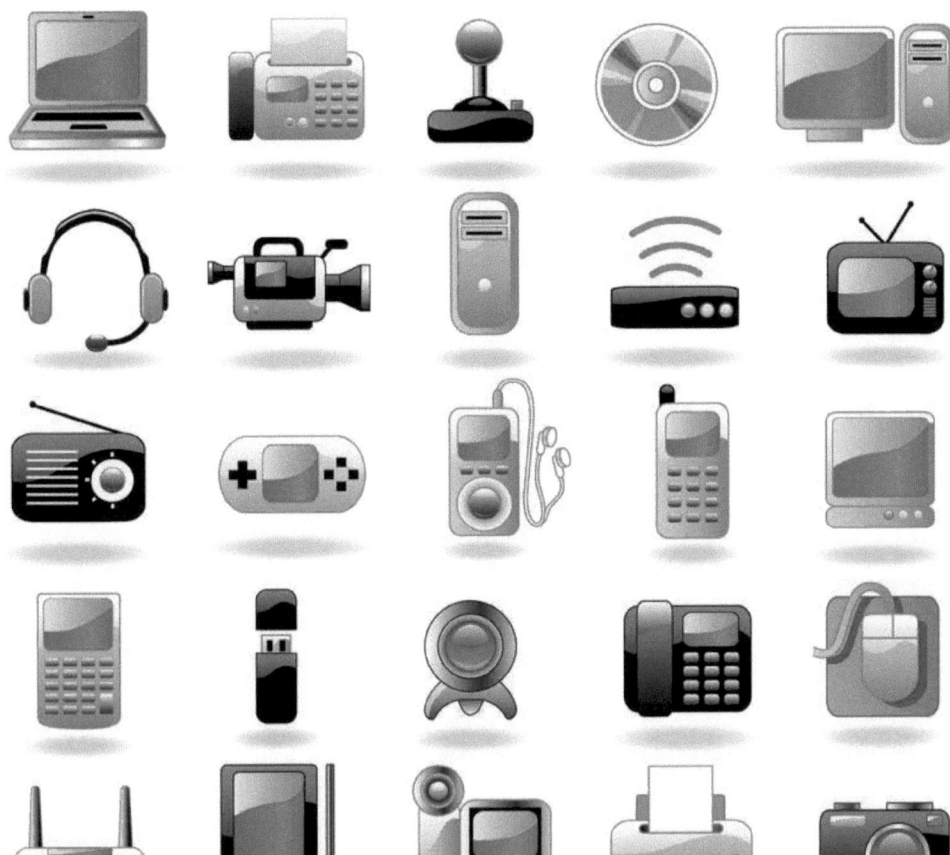

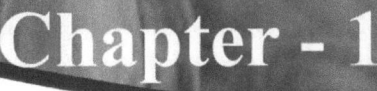

INTRODUCTION TO ELECTRONICS

What is Electronics?

Electronics is a branch of Physics which helps us in understanding various electronic devices.

Dictionary definition – *The science and technology of electric phenomenon is called electronics.* Under electronics, we learn various electric as well as electronic devices.

Difference between Electrical and Electronic Devices

Electrical – This term relates to devices which run on electricity and are used in our day to day lives. For example, toaster, hair dryer, heater, radio, television, etc.

Electronic – This term relates to devices which help in the construction of electrical devices. Resistors, capacitors, amplifiers and transistors are electronic devices which are used in electronic circuits of gadgets like heater, radio, etc.

What Constitutes Electronics?

The study of electronics covers electronic components like capacitors, resistors, inductors, diodes, transistors, etc. and different types of circuits.

An electronic component is a physical entity or an object which is used in an electric circuit.

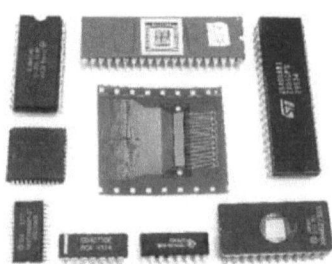

These electric circuits are used in electronic devices like radios, calculators, heaters, electric iron, etc.

An electric circuit is a network of electronic components which is connected to each other keeping in mind various principles, laws and theories of electricity.

Uses of Electronic Components

- These are used in the manufacturing of simple gadgets like basic radio, calculator, hand held video game, etc.
- These are used in making electrical equipments like television, refrigerator, computer, etc.

In the following chapters, we will be reading and learning about electronic devices like –

- Transistor
- Transformer
- Capacitor
- Amplifier
- Resistor

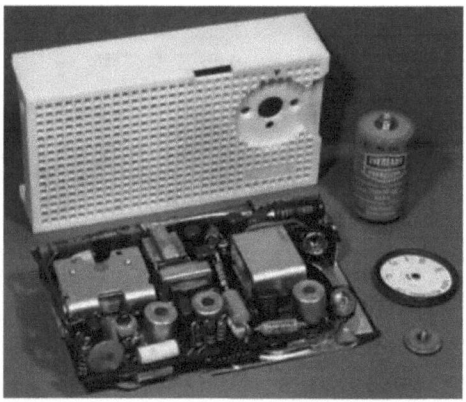

Quick Facts

Some exciting inventions in electronics:

- 1600 – William Gilbert coined the term, 'electricity'.
- 1733 – Benjamin Franklin named the two types of charges as 'positive' and 'negative'.
- 1800 – Alessandro Volta invented an electric battery.
- 1821 – Michael Faraday invented an electric motor.
- 1883 – Electric transformer was invented.
- 1907 – Lee De Forest invented the electric amplifier.
- 1947 – Transistor was invented.

Chapter - 2

ELECTRIC CHARGE AND ELECTRIC CURRENT

Electric Charge

Electric charge is a *physical property of matter*. When matter comes in contact with a charged particle, it experiences a force. This is because it goes through an attraction or repulsion between the electric charge present inside it and the charge it comes in contact with.

Electric Charge is of Two Types:

- Positive charge
- Negative charge

Positive Charge	Negative Charge	Result
+	-	Attraction
+	+	Repulsion
-	-	Repulsion
-	+	Attraction

When two opposite charges come in contact with each other, they experience **attraction**. This is called an *attractive charge*.

For example, a positively charged matter coming in contact with a negatively charged matter experiences an attractive force.

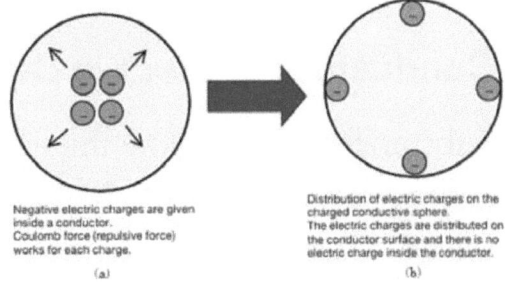

When two similar charges come in contact with each other, they experience **repulsion**. This is called a *repulsive charge*.

For example, positively charged matter coming in contact with another positively charged matter experiences a repulsive force.

Unit

The SI unit of an electric charge is **coulomb**. It is denoted by a capital **'C'**.

Electric Current

Flow of electric charge through a medium is called electric current. An electric current is generated when *electrons move through a conductor, like wire*. It is very similar to water flowing through a pipe.

When electrons continuously move through a conductor, such as wire, electric current is generated. This electric current, or simply called current, is used to run various electronic devices like tube light, fan, motor, microwave, refrigerator, etc.

Unit

The SI unit of electric current is **ampere**. It is denoted by a capital **'A'**.

Ampere = 1 coulomb per second

The amount of electric current is measured using an **ammeter**.

Conductors of Electric Current

Substances which allow the flow of electric charge (or electrons) in themselves are called conductors of electric current.

Good Conductors – Most metals like copper, aluminium, iron are good conductors of electricity. Graphite being a non-metal is also a good conductor of electric current.

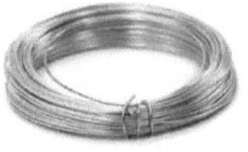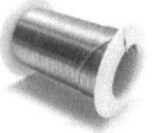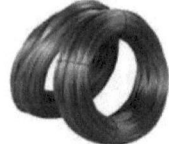

Bad Conductors – Most non-metals like wood, glass, rubber, etc are bad conductors of electric current.

Electric energy is easily transportable via integrated electric grids. After transportation, electric energy is converted into mechanical energy, thermal energy, light energy, chemical energy, etc.

Quick Facts

- When an electric charge builds up on the surface of an object, it creates static electricity.
- Electricity is by no means a purely human invention, and may be observed in several forms in nature, such as lightning.
- A generator is a device that converts mechanical energy into electrical energy. The process is based on the relationship between magnetism and electricity.

- Electric eels can produce strong electric shocks of around 500 volts for both self defence and hunting.
- Electric energy is an intermediate form of energy. It is produced in thermal power stations (where fuel oil, gas, coal, biomass, etc. are burnt), in hydroelectric power stations and nuclear power stations. Smaller quantities are produced by wind, photovoltaic solar panels, sea tides, etc.
- Demand for solar electric energy has consistently grown by 20-25% per year over the past 20 years.
- In 1791, Luigi Galvani published his discovery of bioelectricity, demonstrating that electricity was the medium by which nerve cells passed signals to the muscles.
- In 1882, water was used to electrify two paper mills and a house on the Fox River. The Fox River is a tributary of the Illinois River in the United States. This was the first application of hydroelectric energy.

Chapter - 3

TRANSISTOR

Transistor is a very basic and essential device in most of the electronic devices. A transistor is a semiconductor device which is used to *amplify* and *switch* electronic signals.

Working of a Transistor

Transistors have two main functions – *amplifying* and *switching*.

Transistor as an Amplifier

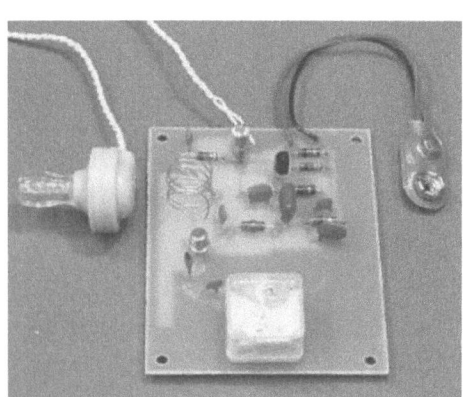

A transistor works as a gatekeeper for current in an electronic device. It is made up of three parts – a base, a collector and an emitter. The collector is like an inlet of the current flow to the base. The base acts as a gate to the flow of electric current. It regulates the current and sends the regulated current to the emitter.

This whole process is similar to using a tap to control the flow of water supplied from the main pipes.

Transistor as a Switch

A transistor works in the same way as an amplifier by regulating the flow of current. After regulating the amount, it makes sure that a specific amount of electric current goes out through the emitter. If the amount of current is equal to the specified amount, the transistor 'switches-on'. If the amount of current is less than the specified amount, the transistor 'switches-off'.

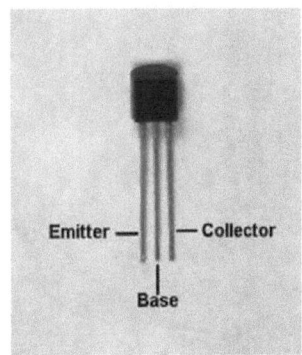

Did You Know?

John Bardeen, Walter Brattain and William Shockley are the scientists who invented the transistor in the year, 1947.

Advantages of Using a Transistor

A transistor is a fundamental unit of modern electronic devices. Devices like radio, calculators, computers, telephones, etc use transistors.

Mass Produced – Good quality transistors can be produced in very large quantities.

Low Cost – Because of their mass production, transistors are very inexpensive.

Flexibility – Transistors are preferred for writing computer programs than to design complex functions in computers.

Quick Facts

- **Semiconductor** – A semiconductor is a substance which allows the flow of electric current under specific conditions. Thus, it is useful in regulating the electric current.
- **Amplify** – The term, 'amplify' means to increase strength.
- The first commercial device to use the transistor was the Sonotone 1010 hearing aid.
- Early transistors were used to amplify audio signals.
- The first transistor radio went on the market in 1954 and had only four transistors.
- Gordon Moore, co-founder of Intel, predicted that the number of transistors on a chip would double about every two years. This is known as Moore's Law.

Chapter - 4

TRANSFORMER

A transformer is an electronic device which is used to *transfer electric current from one circuit to another*.

Electric Current

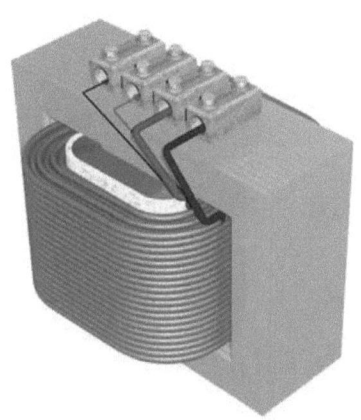

The electricity you get in your house comes to you through a big transformer. The electricity board transmits electric current through wires to a transformer in your residential area. This transformer then distributes the electricity to each and every house of the area. If there was no transformer, the electric current coming straight from electricity board to your house would be very high and would destroy the electric circuit in your house. Then you won't be able to run a tube light or a fan.

Construction of a Transformer

A transformer is a device made up of an *insulated metal core* (usually iron). The two parallel arms of the iron core are coiled with copper wires. These two coils are called primary and secondary winding.

Working of a Transformer

Primary winding of the transformer gets the input voltage which is converted from low voltage to high voltage or vice-versa. To convert low voltage to high voltage, the coils in the secondary windings are increased. To convert high voltage to low voltage, the coils in the secondary windings are decreased.

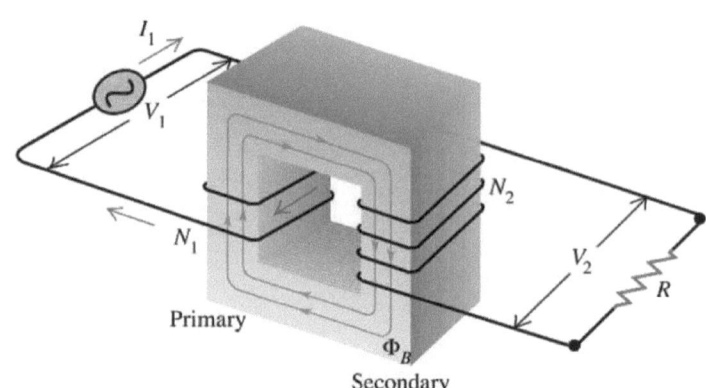

Did You Know?

William Stanley designed the first transformer in the year, **1885**.

Uses of a Transformer

- Transformers modify electric current under difficult conditions like low voltage to high voltage, high voltage to low, etc.
- They distribute electricity over long distances.
- They protect electronic devices from a huge load of electric current.
- They lower the main voltage to a usable level for an electronic device.
- They filter out any problem in the conductor.

Quick Facts

- Voltage, also known as electric tension, is the energy required to move electric current from one point to another. It is measured in 'volts' and is denoted by a capital 'V'.
- Generally, a voltage of 220V is required to run electric equipments
- A circuit is a path between the start point and the end point of the flow of electric current.
- Basically, a transformer is an electrical device used to transfer an alternating current or voltage from one electric circuit to another by the means of electromagnetic induction.

Chapter - 5

CAPACITOR

A capacitor is an electronic device used for *storing electrical energy*.

Construction of a Capacitor

A capacitor is made up of *two conducting plates*, usually metals, at two ends and a non-conducting plate called a 'dielectric' in between them.

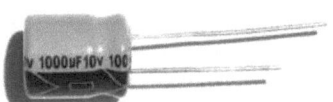

Working of a Capacitor

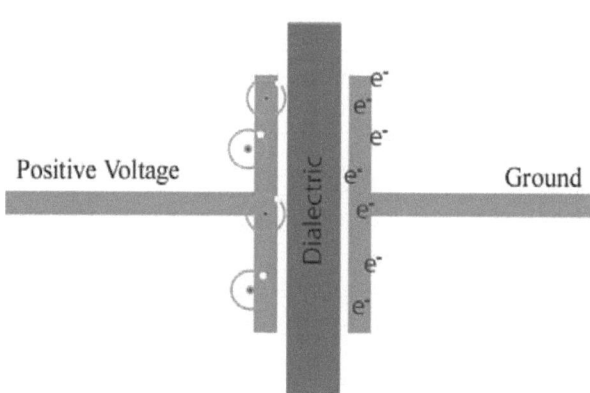

When there is a **voltage fluctuation** across the conductors in a capacitor, an electric field appears across the **dielectric**. This causes positive charge to collect on one conductor and negative charge on another conductor. The energy generated is thus stored in this **electric field**.

Uses of a Capacitor

- Capacitors are widely used in electric circuits of many electrical devices.
- They are used in filter networks for the smooth flow of power supplies.
- They are used in circuits inside a radio to tune into the desired FM station.

Make Your Own Capacitor

Things Required – copper wire, wire strippers, cling film, aluminium foil, cellotape and scissors.

Procedure:

1. Take two pieces of copper wires. Remove 2 cm of plastic covering from the copper wire using wire stripper.
2. Place a piece of cling film on the table. Make sure there isn't any wrinkle.
3. Place a piece of aluminium foil 1cm shorter than the cling film.
4. Attach the end of the stripped copper wire on the aluminium foil with the help of a cellotape. The copper wire and the aluminium foil must remain in contact with each other.
5. Now place another piece of cling film on the aluminium foil. Repeat steps 2 to 4 again.
6. Roll the whole thing into a cylinder with cling film on the outside.
7. Put the cellotape on the cylinder in order to hold all things together.
8. Now the aluminium foil acts as a *conductor* and the cling film as a *dielectric*.

Quick Facts

- A dielectric is another term used for insulators/bad conductors of electric current.
- An electric field is a virtual space surrounding the electrically charged particles.
- The concept of electric field was introduced by Michael Faraday.
- Capacitors contain a circuit, light and a switch. Because of the ability of the capacitor to block current flow, it is often used as a filter.
- A capacitor cannot produce new electrons. A capacitor can only store the electrons.
- The unit of capacitance is called a farad. A 1-farad capacitor is able to store one coulomb of charge at one volt.
- Super capacitors are electric double layer capacitors which have a capacitance of 0.47 Farad.

Chapter - 6

INDUCTOR

An inductor is a two-terminal electronic device which is used to store energy in a magnetic field. It is also known as a **reactor** or a **coil**. It is a basic component which is used in devices where voltage and current change.

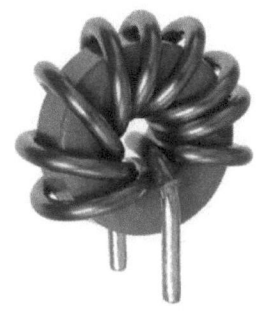

Construction of an Inductor

An inductor is a coil of conducting material (such as copper wire) wound on a permanently magnetised iron core.

Working of an Inductor

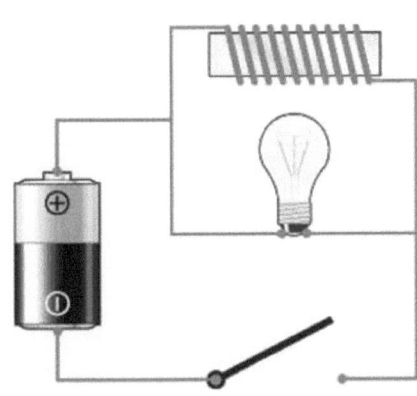

An inductor is simply a wire coil wrapped on a magnetised iron core. It opposes the flow of electric current. When a voltage is applied to a coil of wire, a magnetic field is created around the coils. This magnetic field gives birth to an opposing **voltage**. As voltage is the process of flow of electric current, therefore, the inductor opposes this current.

Uses of an Inductor

- Large inductors are used in power supplies.
- Small inductors are used in circuits used in radio reception and transmission.
- They are used to decrease the voltage from lightning strikes.
- They are used to limit faulty currents in a device.

Make Your Own Inductor

Things Required:

A copper wire, 6 inches long, a bar magnet, an iron nail

Procedure:

1. A bar magnet has two magnetic poles at its two ends – south and north. Decide which polarity you want to give your iron nail.
2. Place the iron nail horizontally on the table. Gently rub one end of the bar magnet from head of the nail to its tail.
3. Repeat this action continuously for 5-10 minutes with the same end of the magnet.
4. Now, start winding the copper wire on the middle of the nail tightly.
5. Your inductor is ready.

Quick Facts

- A magnetised iron core is that which has been made permanently magnetic in nature by keeping in contact with a magnetic field for a long time.
- The inductor stores electrical energy in the form of magnetic energy.
- The inductor does not allow Alternating Current (AC) to flow through it, but does allow Direct Current (DC) to flow through it.
- Typical applications for inductors used in power supply circuits are "voltage conversion" and "choke," and these inductors are used in a wide range of electronic equipment.
- Inductors store electrical energy in magnetic fields.
- They act as open circuit at first when we apply DC (Direct Current) to them, but after a while, they freely allow it to pass.
- They oppose to changes in current.

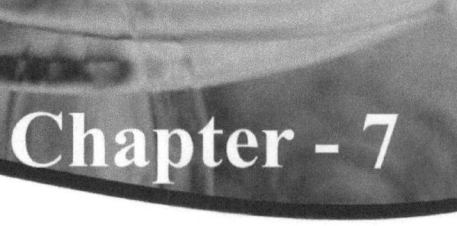

Chapter - 7

RESISTOR

Resistors are very common elements of electronic circuits and electrical networks. A resistor is a device which opposes the flow of electric current in a circuit. It controls and impedes the passage of current.

Unit

Resistors offer resistance to a device. This property is measured in Ohm. It is symbolised as 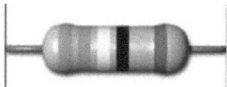 .

Construction of a Resistor

A basic resistor is made up of powdered carbon bound by an adhesive like glue. It has two metal wires at both ends of its cylindrical body.

Did You Know?

The coloured stripes on the body of a resistor help in calculating the value of that resistor.

Working of a Resistor

A resistor works to break the flow of current in a device. Let's understand this with the help of an example. Imagine water flowing through a pipe. If we decrease the diameter of the mouth of the pipe, the amount of water flowing out would decrease. If we increase the pressure of water, then it would generate some amount of heat.

Types of Resistors

Fixed resistors – These are resistors whose values are fixed.

Variable resistors – These are resistors whose values can be increased or decreased while connected to a circuit.

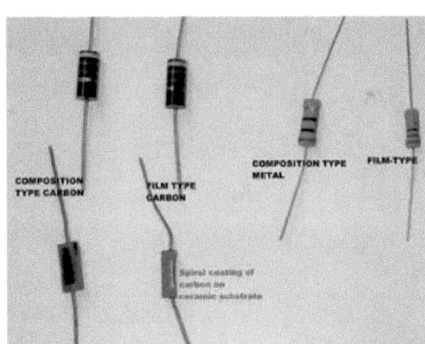

Types of Resistors

Uses of a Resistor

- They are used in television and radio circuits.
- They are used as heating elements in heaters, irons, toasters, etc.
- They are used as filaments in light bulbs.

Make your own Resistor

Things required – A pencil, knife/cutter, two pieces of 6-inch copper wire, soldering iron, a nail (same thickness as of the pencil lead), a wooden board.

Procedure

1. Remove the lead from the pencil with the help of a knife/cutter. Be careful while doing this.
2. Fix a nail on a wooden board.
3. Take a piece of copper wire. Tightly wind a 2 inches wire on the nail.

4. Your wire will get a spiral shape. Repeat the above step with the second wire.
5. Now insert one end of the pencil lead into the spiral part of the copper wire. Bind it with the help of solder iron.
6. Repeat the above step with the second piece of copper wire on the other end of the lead.
7. Your resistor is ready.

Quick Facts

- Resistors are used to create a known voltage to the current ratio in an electric circuit.
- The higher the value of resistance which is measured in ohms, the lower the current will be.
- Resistors are colour coded. Look for the colour stripe on the resistor indicating which way the current is flowing. The power flows from the end without the stripe to the end with the stripe.
- The Ohm's Law states that the potential difference between the two points on a resistor and the current flowing through it must be proportional. The electrical resistance is equal to the voltage drop across the resistor divided by the current through the resistor.

Chapter - 8

USES OF ELECTRONICS

Since the beginning of the modern age, the world has seen many great inventions in the field of science and technology. The advent of electricity is one of many such great inventions. The electric and electronic devices we use today are based on these inventions. These devices have become important and significant parts of our 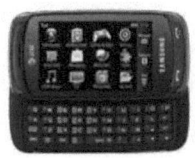 life. Today, we can't imagine our lives without these gadgets as they have become indispensable for us.

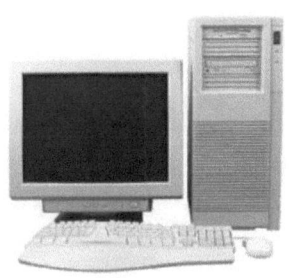

In the above chapters, we have read about many small and basic electronic devices like *transistors, transformers, capacitors, amplifiers and resistors*. These are mere components for the production of gadgets like radio, computer, television, cell phones, etc. But, without them, these gadgets don't have any foundation.

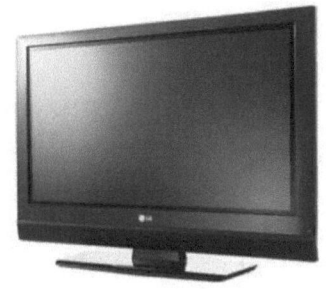

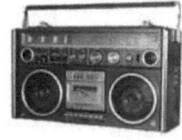

Let us learn some important and significant uses of electronic devices.

Communication

Electronic devices like radio, television, internet, phones, etc are the biggest and popular means of communication today. These devices and gadgets help us connect with the world at large.

Medical Health

Electronic devices find their way in modern day medical health care through machines like *MRI, CAT, CT scan, X-ray scan*, etc. Electronic equipments like pacemakers are a gift to the humans by electronic technology.

Transportation

Vehicles like *aeroplanes, helicopters, metro, bullets* and such new age transport mediums use electric and electronic technologies. This ensures better speed and comfort at low cost, while saving the time of transportation.

Research & Development

Fibre optical, nano technology, wireless technology – all these had their basis on electronic components. Development of spacecrafts, satellites and other new techniques requires the help of electronic technology.

Electronic Trading

With the advent of *internet, electronic trading* has developed at a very fast pace. People use internet for trading, and they use credit and debit cards for shopping.

Entertainment

People use mobile phones, digital cameras, music players, laptops, television, etc. to entertain themselves. Electronic devices have made life much more enjoyable than before.

General Use

From a remote control to a coffee grinder, electronic devices are making their presence felt at every step of our lives. Today, they are a part of our daily routine.

Quick Facts

- Electronics are the basis of many modern technologies, from hi-fl systems to missile control systems.
- Electronics are systems that control things by automatically switching tiny electrical circuits on and off.
- Transistors are electronic switches. They are made of materials called semiconductors that change their ability to conduct electricity.
- Diodes are transistors with two connectors. They control an electric current by switching it on or off.
- Triodes are transistors with three connectors that amplify the electric current (make it bigger) or reduce it.
- A silicon chip is thousands of transistors linked together by thin metal strips in an integrated circuit, on a single crystal of the semi-conductor, silicon.
- The electronic areas of a chip are those treated with traces of chemicals, such as boron and phosphorus, which alter the conductivity of silicon.

Chapter - 9

INTRODUCTION TO COMMUNICATION

What is Communication?

Communication is a process by which a person can deliver his message to another person.

The term, 'communication' is derived from the Latin word, *communis*, which means 'to share'.

We use communication to express our views and opinions and listen to other's views and opinions. Communication is also a process through which we send across important information and receive a feedback.

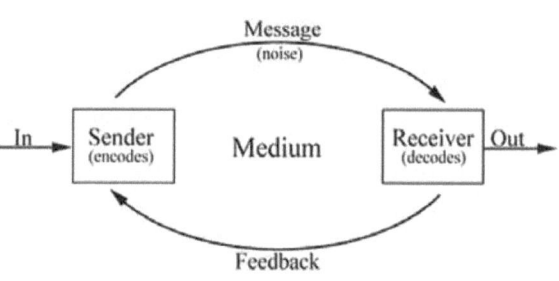

Elements of Communication:

- **Sender** – A person or a group of persons who wants to communicate or send a message

- **Message** – A piece of information which needs to be shared
- **Receiver** – A person or group of persons to whom the message is directed

We communicate through following mediums:
- Speaking
- Through body language
- Writing letters
- Telephone
- Newspapers
- Radio
- Television
- Internet

Beginning of Communication

The need to express himself/herself to others is one of the main needs of a human being, apart from air, water and food.

Since the evolution of the earth, man has tried to communicate with others through various ways. When there was no language, man tried to communicate through gestures and sounds. Later, he used pictures and drawings to communicate. Some of the pictographs found in archaeological sites of Mesopotamian and Indus Valley Civilization are perfect examples of man's efforts to express himself.

The advent of language made it easier for the early man to express himself. He could now communicate easily. The invention of grammar and scripts made it all the more easier for him to write and express.

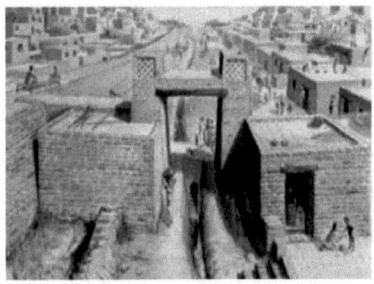
The Indus Valley Civilization

Since then, the world has seen the advent

of hundreds of languages and many mediums of communication. Today, a person sitting in one corner of the world can get in touch with a person in the opposite corner of the world within moments. Science and technological advancement has made the process of communication a very easy process.

Quick Facts

- Early modern communication took place in three main modes: spoken words, manuscript writing, especially letters and the print. Oral communication was the oldest of these three.
- Beginning from the Renaissance, writing developed as an important form of personal expression, particularly among the educated and the upper classes.
- Posts and Telegraphs, Telephone, Fax, Pagers, E-mail and Chatting (through Internet) are some of the modern means of communication.
- Radio and Television, Newspapers and Cinema are some of the modern means of mass communication in the present world.

Chapter - 10

TYPES OF COMMUNICATIONS

Communication means to contact others and to send and receive messages. We express ourselves through speaking, writing and indicating.

Communication through speech is called *verbal communication*.

Communication through writing and indicating is called *non-verbal communication*.

The different mediums through which we send our messages are called communication systems.

The two types of communication systems are:
- Personal Communication
- Mass Communication

Personal Communication

The process through which we send and receive messages and information to and from an individual is called personal communication.

For example, writing a letter to your friend or speaking to your relative on a phone. Also,

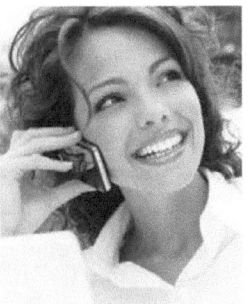

e-mailing and chatting on internet with a person is a part of personal communication.

Following mediums are used in personal communication:

- Post
- Telegraph
- Telephone
- E-mail and Internet

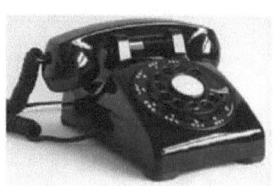
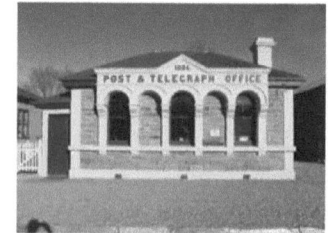

Advantages of Personal Communication:

- We can communicate directly with the person we want to communicate.
- It gives us flexibility of time and place. We can talk on phone or mobile from anywhere.
- It gives us privacy.

Mass Communication

The process through which we send messages and information to a large group of people (or masses) is called mass communication. It doesn't give information to one person, but to the community at large.

For example, a newsreader reading news on radio and television.

The following mediums are used in mass communication:

- Newspapers and Magazines
- Radio
- Television
- Internet

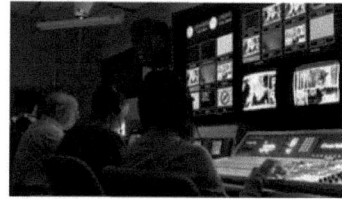

Means of Mass Communication

Mass communication is divided into:

- **Print Communication** – Newspapers, magazines, leaflets, pamphlets, brochures, etc.

- **Electronic Communication** – Radio, Television and Internet.

Advantages of Mass Communication:

- They are very useful for sending information to a very large group of people.
- Everyone gets the information almost at the same time.
- Has a very low cost as compared to the personal means of communication.

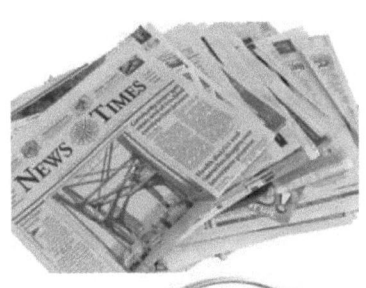
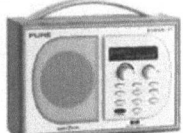

Quick Facts

- Based on the style and purpose of communication, there can be two broad categories: Formal and Informal Communication, that have their own set of characteristic features.
- Formal Communication includes all the instances where communication has to occur in a set formal format. Typically, this can include all sorts of business or corporate communication.
- Informal Communication includes instances of free and unrestrained conversation between people who share a casual rapport with each other, such as friends, family members, etc.
- Even though the whole process of communication may seem so simple, the effectiveness of each type depends to a great extent on certain internal and external environmental factors and also the communicator's ability to send, receive, decode and send a response.

Chapter - 11

POST AND TELEGRAPH

Post and Telegraph are very important means of personal communication.

Before the advent of the modern means of communications like telephone, radio, television and internet, letters and other means of postal communications were the only significant media of personal communication.

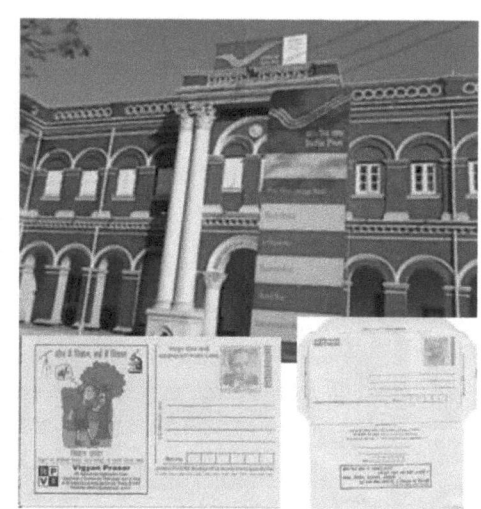

Did You Know?

The **Indian Post Office** was set up in the year, **1854**.

How does a postal system work?

The process of postal system starts as soon as you dispatch your properly addressed letter (including the postal/pin/zip code) in a letter box. The letters and posts from these public letter boxes get collected into a post office, where they are sorted into different stacks according to their post codes. Then these posts and letters are dispatched to different regions. Once your letter reaches to the post office of the specified office, a postman collects it and delivers it in your correspondent's address.

Postal Service in India

In India, the Department of Posts is a government-operated postal service. The Indian Postal Service is the most widely used postal service in the world. There are around 1,55,333 post offices in our country.

The Indian Postal Service was first established under the East India Company, during the British rule, under the name, Company Mail in 1688. The possession of the postal service was given to the Indian Post Office in the year, 1854.

Stamps

The *adhesive stamps* were first introduced on October 1, 1854 in India. These were the first in Asia.

Types of Postal Services

International Registered Post – It is sent when the sender wishes to have a receipt of the mail from the receiver.

Speed Post – It is sent when the sender wants the mail to reach the next day, anywhere in the country.

Parcels – It is used for sending parcels upto 35 kg anywhere in the country.

Quick Facts

- Post or Postal Codes are specific codes given to each area of a city/town in every region of a country. A post code makes it easier for your post to reach the desired place conveniently and on time.
- The highest post office of the world is at a height of about 15,500 feet in Hikkim, Himachal Pradesh.
- In 2011, the Indian Postal Service inaugurated a floating post office in the Dal Lake, Srinagar, Jammu & Kashmir.
- At the time of independence of India, there were about 23,344 post offices, which were primarily in urban areas.
- As of March 31, 2011, the Indian Postal Service has been recorded to have 154,866 post offices, of which 139,040 (89.78%) are in rural areas and around 15,826 (10.22%) in urban areas. It has about 25,464 departmental POs and 129,402 ED BPOs.
- The U.S. Postal Service is the core of the trillion dollar mailing industry that employs more than 8 million people.

Chapter - 12

TELEPHONE

The word, 'telephone' is made up of two words, *tele* meaning 'distance' and *phonetics* meaning sound. Thus, Telephone means *sound from a distance*.

How Does a Telephone Work?

Process - A telephone consists of a microphone which converts the sound waves into electric current and sends it through a telephone network to another phone. The earphone or speaker in the receiving phone converts this electric signal back into sound wave.

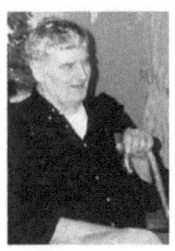

Did You Know?

Alexander Graham Bell was the first person to invent a telephone, in the year **1876**.

Advent of Telephones

In the beginning, there was only one kind of telephone – *a fixed cable handset with a receiver and a body with a dial* pad. It is known as 'Landline' today. As the technology progressed, a new kind of phone came into being – a cordless phone.

George Sweigert, in **1966**, invented the **cordless phone** – a portable phone without a cable. It consisted of a handset with speaker/receiver and a base station. This phone could be carried around within a specified range of the base station. This provided tremendous flexibility to the user. The only drawback was that it needed to be plugged into the base for charging.

Then in **1973**, **Dr. Martin Cooper** of **Motorola** came out with the first mobile phone of the history. This is hailed as one of the biggest resolution in the field of telecommunication. Today, almost every person carries a mobile phone.

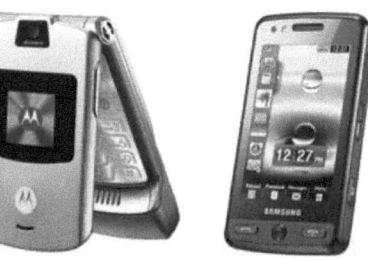

Telephone Services in India

Today, there are around *33.19 million landline phones in India. India is world's second largest mobile phone using nation with over 881 million users, in 2011.* Also, it is the world's third largest internet using nation with over 121 million users, in 2011.

Today with the arrival of smart phones, people have got most of the telecommunication features in their handset. A smart phone has features like internet surfing, e-mailing, chat, message texting, etc.

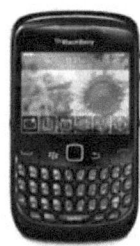

Advantages of Telephone:

- It is the easiest mode of personal communication today.
- With the advent of mobile phones, telecommunications have left behind all the other modes of communications as the most frequently used communication medium.

Quick Facts

- The first cellular phone network was established in the United States in the year, 1983.
- Our telephone is made up of 201 parts, every one of which had to be planned, produced and assembled with an unusual degree of accuracy.
- As a tribute to Alexander Graham Bell when he died in 1922, all the telephones stopped ringing for one full minute.
- The great author and writer, Mark Twain was one of the first to have a phone in his home.
- Alexander Graham Bell thought the phone should be answered with "Hoy, Hoy" instead of "Hello".
- In 1956 the first transatlantic telephone cable was placed on the ocean floor and rests as deep as 12,000 feet! It runs from Newfoundland, Canada to Scotland!
- There are about 149,084,370 telephone lines in the world and thousands more are being added every day.

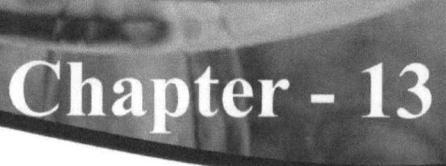

Chapter - 13

NEWSPAPERS AND MAGAZINES

Newspapers were the earliest means of mass communication. Newspapers and Magazines also come under the *print communication*.

Newspapers

Around the world, newspapers are the most sought after means of communication for all the information regarding national events, political news, sports, science, technology, economics, business and trade, current affairs, etc.

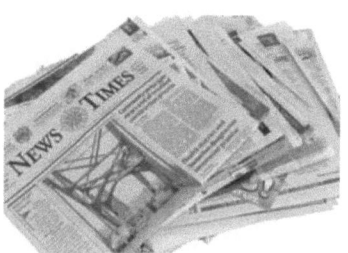

Newspapers are divided into:

- **National Dailies** – Newspapers which are circulated throughout the country are called national dailies. For example, *Hindustan Times, The Times of India, Indian Express,* etc in English and *Hindustan, Navbharat Times, Dainik Bhaskar,* etc in Hindi.

- **Regional Newspapers** – Newspapers which are circulated within a specific region are called regional newspapers. For example, *The Hindu* in south India, *Dainik Jagran* in north India, etc.

- **Tabloids** – Newspapers which are not circulated in the morning, but are circulated during the noon or evening are called tabloids. For example, *Mail Today, Afternoon Despatch & Courier, Mid Day*, etc.

The Bengal Gazette was the first newspaper to be published in India, in the year, 1780, in Calcutta (Kolkata).

Did You Know?

By the year, 2007, there were around 6580 daily newspapers being published across the world.

Magazines

Apart from newspapers, magazines constitute a large share of the print communication. In India, around *75 popular magazines are published every year*. Magazines are generally based on the following subjects:

- Current affairs
- Politics
- Business
- Economics
- Science and technology
- Sports
- Entertainment
- Lifestyle

Journals

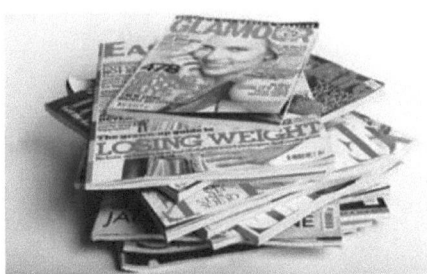

Magazines

Also magazines are circulated *periodically*, unlike newspapers. Based on the periodicity, magazines are divided into the following:

- Weekly – Published every week
- Fortnightly – Published every 15 days
- Monthly – Published every month
- Quarterly – Published every three months
- Annually – Published once a year

Advantages of Newspapers and Magazines:

- They have a longer shelf life than television or radio. It means that people can keep their copy of newspaper/magazine with them and read or refer it again whenever they want to.
- They have greater reach in the local difficult terrain where radio or television signals don't reach.

Quick Facts

- The Newspaper began its roots as early as Julius Caesar times. During that time, it was regarded as those scrolls read in front of the public to inform them of important happenings and events. Its first recorded account was as early as 59 B.C. and the name of the first newspaper was Acta Diurna.
- The Gentleman's Magazine, first published in 1731, in London, is considered to have been the first general-interest magazine. Edward Cave, who edited The Gentleman's Magazine under the pen name, 'Sylvanus Urban', was the first to use the term, 'magazine', on the analogy of a military storehouse of varied material, ultimately derived from the Arabic-makhazin ('storehouses') by way of the French language. The oldest consumer magazine still in print is The Scots Magazine, which was first published in 1739.

Chapter - 14

RADIO

Radio is the most basic as well as one of the earliest means of electronic communication. It is the *first wireless communication system in the world*.

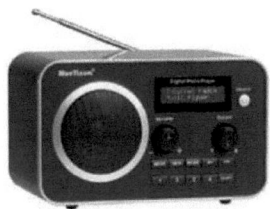
A Modern Radio

How Does a Radio Transmission Work?

Radio transmission uses the concept of electromagnetic waves to send and receive information.

Process – The *sound energy is converted into electrical energy*. This electrical energy is send to a transmitter which converts this electric current into electromagnetic waves. These electromagnetic waves are then transmitted into the atmosphere. A radio set acts as a receiver. The *antenna* in a radio set catches the electromagnetic waves. These waves are then turned into electric current. This electric current is then converted into sound energy which we can hear in the form of *music, news,* etc.

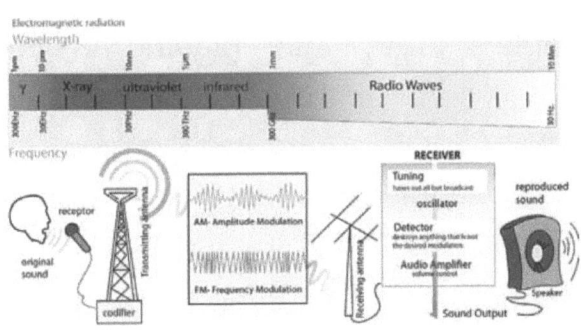

Did You Know?

Guglielmo Marconi of Italy was the first to send and receive the first radio signals in **1895**.

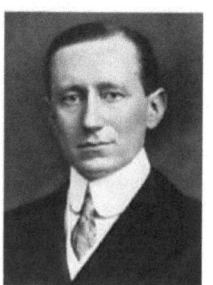

A Radio runs on the following band widths:
- **AM** – Amplitude Modulation
- **FM** – Frequency Modulation

Most of the private radio stations are based on FM.

Radio Broadcasting in India

The *first radio broadcast in India took place on July 23, 1927.*

It was broadcasted by the *Indian Broadcasting Company (IBC)* which inaugurated its *first radio station in Bombay (Mumbai)*.

Bombay (Mumbai), Calcutta (Kolkata), Madras (Chennai) and Bangalore (Bengaluru) were the first few cities to have radio stations in the country.

Today, there are on an average 10 radio stations (mostly FM) in important cities of the country. These stations include private as well as public radio stations.

Advantages of Radio for Mass Communication:
- Radio is a universal medium and can be used at any time.
- It does not have to be viewed or read unlike other mediums. Therefore, it saves people's time while playing in the background.
- People can give their feedback on the content of the program by 'phoning' the radio stations, or by sending sms through their mobiles, by sending e-mails through the Internet.
- Information broadcast through radio can even be useful for the illiterate people.

Quick Facts

- Radio frequencies are between 300 GHz to 3 Hz.
- The Radio waves travel at a speed of about 186,000 miles per second, and were discovered in 1865 by James Clerk Maxwell.
- The All India Radio (AIR) is the government broadcasting body in India.
- FM broadcasting is preferred over AM broadcasting because FM transmissions are not disturbed by static interference. Also, FM transmissions have better sound quality.
- The Radio waves are considered to be Electromagnetic Radiations.
- An Amplitude Modulation (AM) wave is considered to be as long as a football field.
- Edwin Howard Armstrong, a genius by birth invented the Frequency Modulation (FM) band.

Chapter - 15

TELEVISION

Television is the most important medium of electronic communication. The term, 'Television' is made up of the Greek word, *tele* which means 'far' and the Latin word, *visio* which means 'sight'. Thus, television means 'seeing from the distance'.

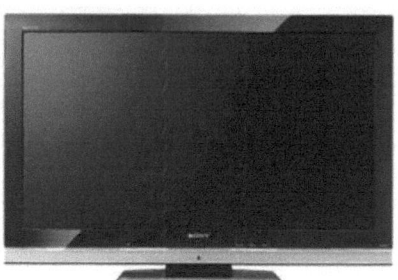

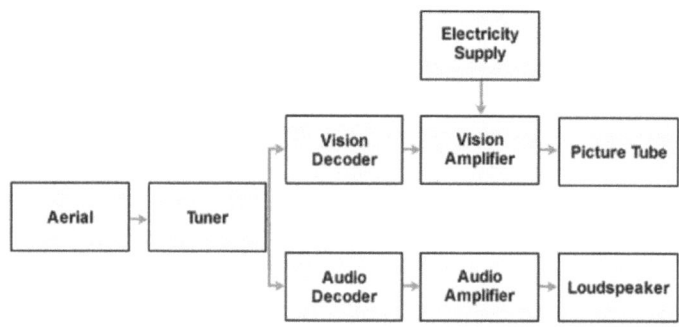

A Television is a telecommunication medium which receives and displays moving images along with the sounds.

How Does a Television Work?

Process - The data (audio-video) is converted into electric signal. This electric signal is then transmitted through a transmitter into the atmosphere. These signals are then received by an antenna which converts them back into audio and video data. This data is then seen and heard on the television screen and speakers.

Did You Know?

Philo Farnsworth of Great Britain transmitted the television image in **1927**.

Television in India

Television is one of the main medium of information as well as entertainment for people. Earlier, there were only two channels on Indian television, i.e., DD National and DD Metro. But today, there is a flood of private channels like Star, Zee, Sony, etc.

There are all kinds of program broadcasted on television like news, entertainment, sports shows, quiz shows, fiction serials, etc.

Advantages of Television:

- Very useful for illiterate people who can take advantage of the fact that it is an audio-visual medium.
- People get latest information and news because of instantaneous transmission services.
- It plays an important part in educating the people on several important issues. Being a visual medium, it has a greater impact on people's thinking.

Quick Facts

- In 1938, the television broadcasts were, for the first time, able to be taped and edited. Prior to that, only live transmission was possible.
- India is the third largest television viewing nation in the world, following China and the United State (US), the US, being the first.
- National telecasts were introduced in India in the year, 1982.
- In 1982, the coloured television sets came into the Indian market.
- In year 1926, J.L. Baird first displayed television which had only 30 lines and gave coarse image. Currently the digital signal of the television sends pictures with 1080 lines.
- A 103-inch plasma TV from Panasonic is the largest plasma TV currently available in the market, costing approximately around $70,000.

Chapter - 16

THE INTERNET

Internet is the latest and most convenient medium of mass communication. The Internet is a worldwide system of interconnected computer networks that uses certain guidelines called the *Internet Protocols* to give information to people across the globe.

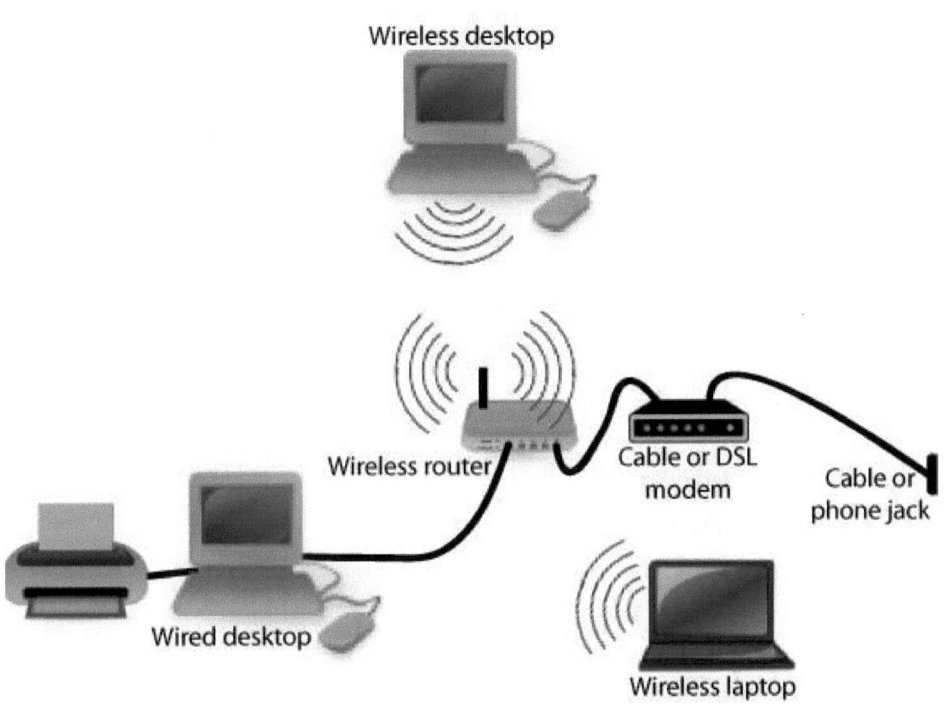

How Does the Internet Work?

Process – The Internet is a huge structure of interconnected computer networks. These networks have a number of computers under them. In a network, computers are connected to a server. A server is a system which receives the information from the *router*. A router is the link between the network and the internet. This router gathers the information from the communication mediums like *telephone lines, satellites, fibre-optic cables,* etc.

Did You Know?

An Internet is a result of the research conducted by the *United States of America in 1960, for the development of computer networks.*

Internet in India

India is the world's fourth largest Internet using nation with over 121 million users in 2011. In the year, **1995**, the **Videsh Sanchar Nigam Ltd. (VSNL)** introduced the Internet in India. By 2005, around 40 million people in the country were regular users of the Internet.

Today, there are around *180 Internet service providing companies in the country,* such as MTNL, VSNL, Airtel, Aircel, Sify, Reliance, Tata, etc.

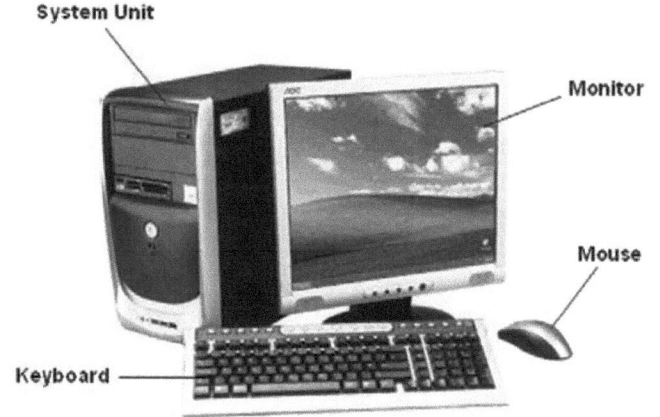

Advantages of the Internet:

- It allows greater flexibility in working hours.
- It can be accessed by a number of mediums like mobile, data cards, etc. It doesn't require a wired network.
- You can have access to almost any information in the world.
- It gives you information, entertainment, latest news, trading platform, shopping platform, e-banking, and many such services.
- *E-mail, chats and social networking* are good platforms for giving out information and being in touch with a large number of people.

Quick Facts

- The World Wide Web (WWW) came into existence in the year, 1994.
- An internet service provider is a company which operates the Internet on various networks like the Local Area Network (LAN) and the World Area Network (WAN).
- The Internet grew at a much faster pace than the Radio and TV as it reached 50 million users in just 5 years, whereas the Radio and TV took 38 and 13 years respectively to reach this target. Out of this, 35.6 percent of internet users are Asian.
- The first webcam was deployed at the Cambridge University computer lab with the sole purpose to monitor a particular coffee maker and hence, avoid wasted trips to an empty pot.

Glossary

Pedalling: To move the pedals of a bicycle

Rickshaws: A man pedalling on a tricycle

Paved: To prepare or make easier

Mast: A structure rising above the hull/upper part of a ship or a boat

Palanquin: A covered litter, formerly used in India, carried on the shoulders of four men

Emission: Radiation

Carriages: A wheeled vehicle for carrying people drawn by horses

Commercial: Suitable or fit for a wide, popular market

Locomotive: A self-propelled, vehicular engine powered by steam, diesel/electricity

Conveyance: A means of communication

Sleigh: Another name for sledge, i.e., a vehicle drawn by horses or dogs

Convenient: Easy, suitable, agreeable

Revenue: The income of a government from taxation, excise duties, customs, etc.

Purview: Range of operation, authority

Concrete: An artificial stone like material

Approved: To consent or agree to

Freight: Transportation of goods by water

Lifeline: A vital line of access or communication

Entities: Things, something having a real existence

Efficiency: Competency

Excessive: Enormous, extravagant

Alternative: A possibility of choice, either of such choices

Frequency: Regularity, periodicity, how often

Hovercraft: A vehicle that can travel across both land and water on a cushion of air

Transit: An act of passing across or through

Consumption: Utilisation, depletion

Amplifier: An electronic device used to increase the strength of signal fed into it

Device: Machine, instrument

Electronic: Concerned with or operated by devices in which electrons are conducted through a body

Fluctuation: Continual change from one point condition to another

Transmission: Transfer, passing of

Impedes: Blocks, thwarts, checks

Insert: To put in or between, introduce

Indispensable: Essential, absolutely necessary

Broad casting: To transmit or relay programmes on radio or television

Modulation: Variation, intonation, transition, inflection

Feedback: Response or reaction

Displays; Shown or exhibits, unfolds
Converts: Transforms, to change, to alter
Interconnected: Interrelated, interlinked
Protocol: A record of data or observations on a particular experiment
Accessed: Judged, verified, adjudged

CAREER & BUSINESS MANAGEMENT
(कॅरियर एण्ड बिजनेस मैनेजमेंट)

JOB RELATED
(नौकरी सम्बन्धी)

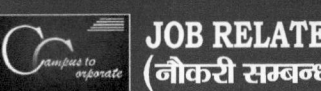

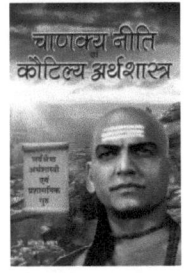 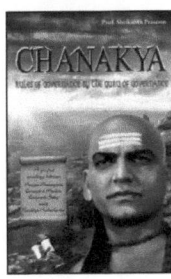 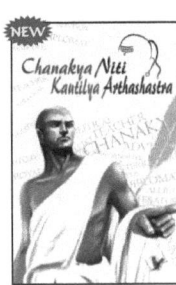 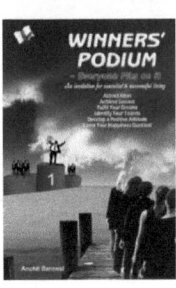 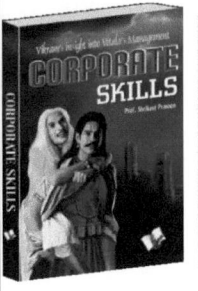 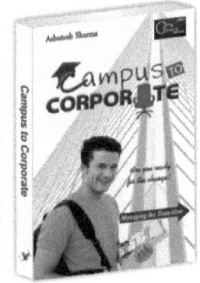

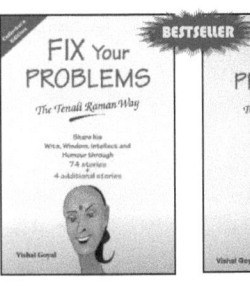 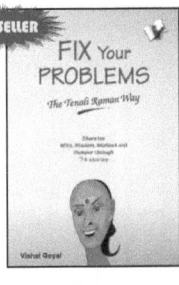 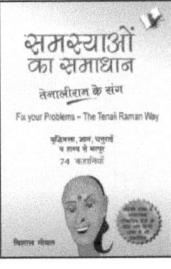 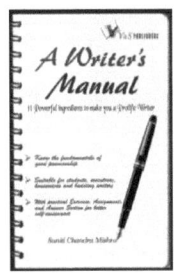 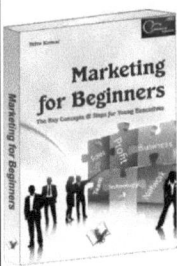 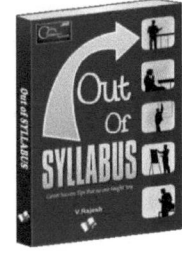

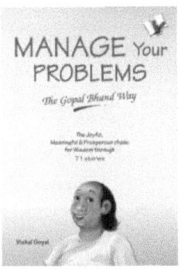 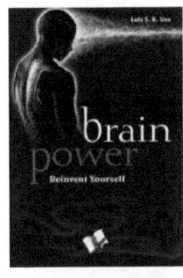 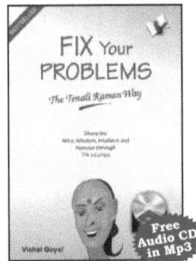 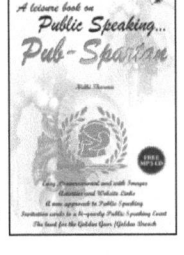 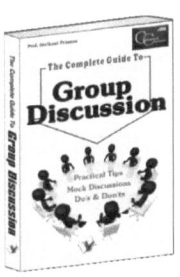 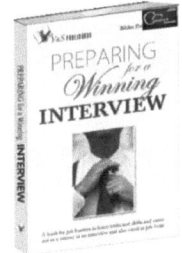

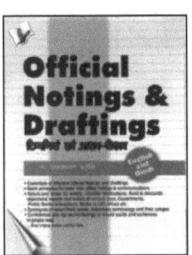 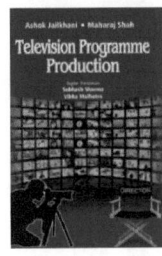 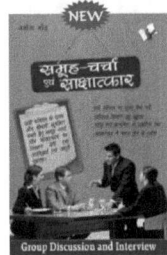 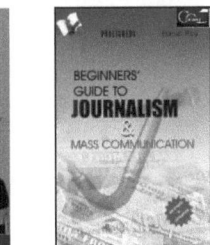 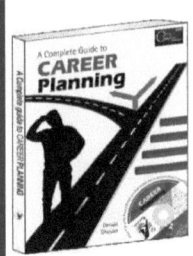 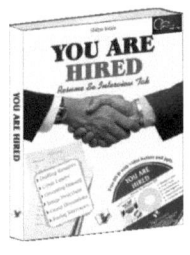

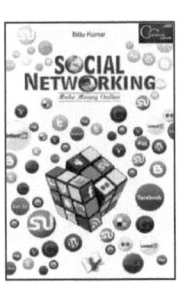 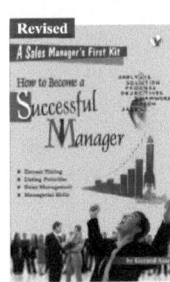 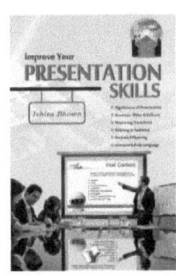 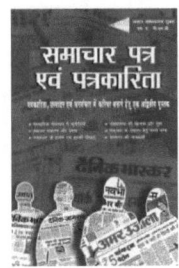 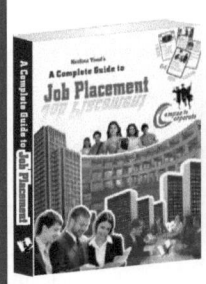 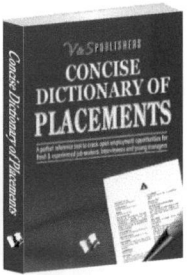

Contact us at sales@vspublishers.com

STUDENT DEVELOPMENT/LEARNING
(छात्र विकास/लर्निंग)

JOKES
(हास्य)

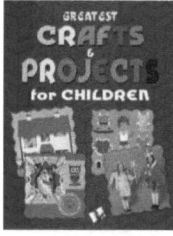 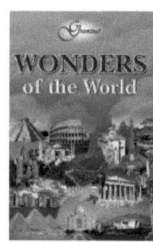 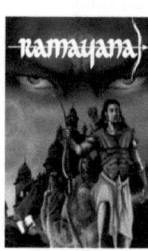 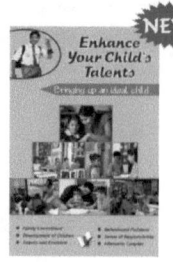 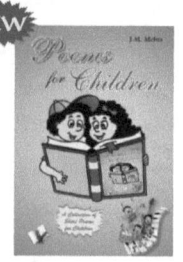 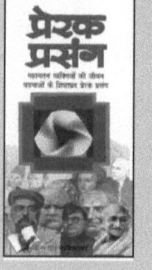 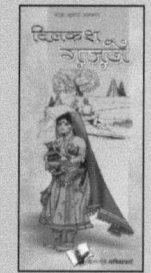

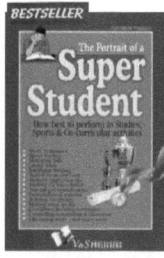 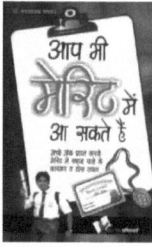 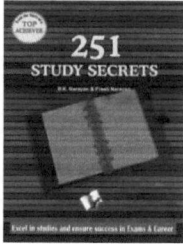 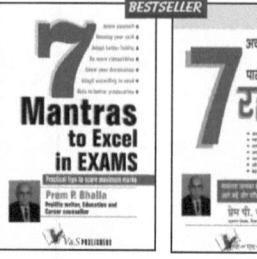 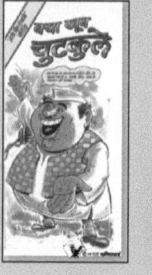 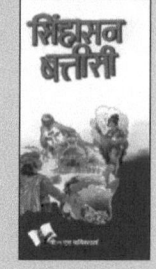

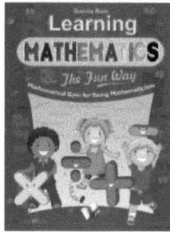 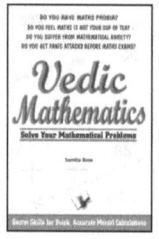 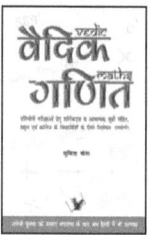 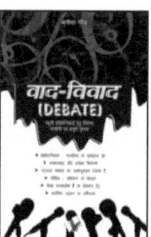 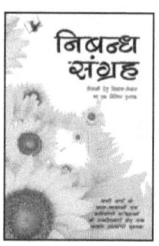 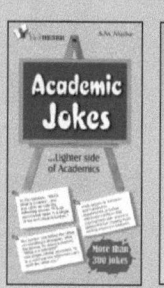 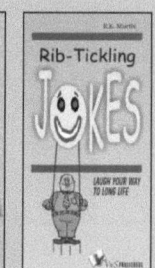

MAGIC & FACT (जादू एवं तथ्य)

MUSIC (संगीत)

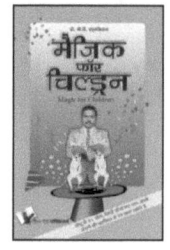 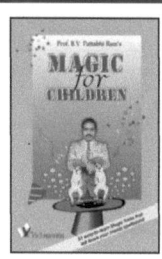 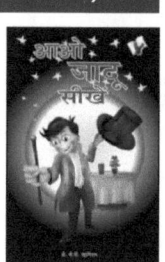 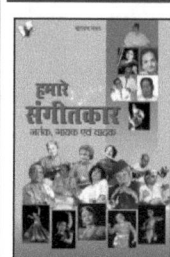 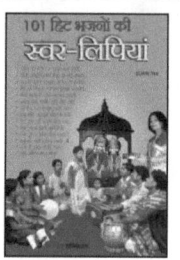 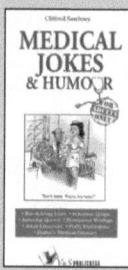 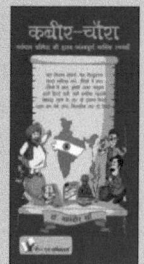

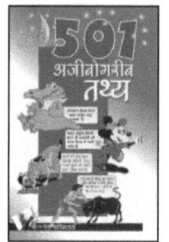 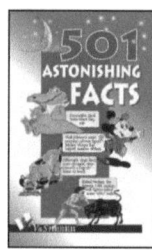 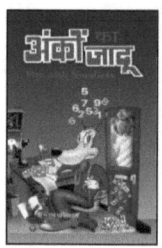

COMPUTER

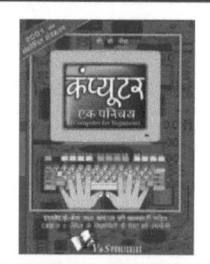 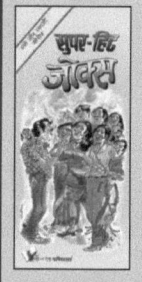 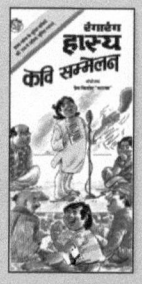 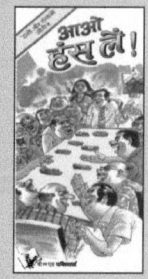

All books available at www.vspublishers.com

Quiz Books (प्रश्नोत्तरी की पुस्तकें)   MYSTERIES (रहस्य)

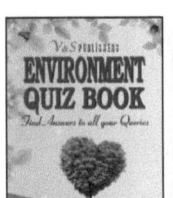 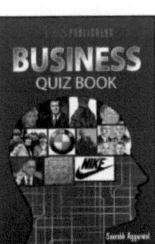 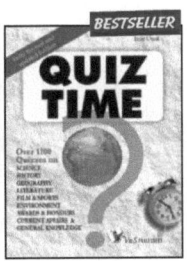 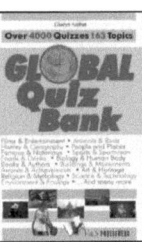 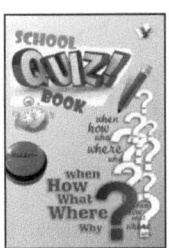 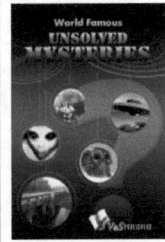 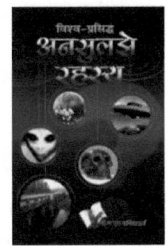

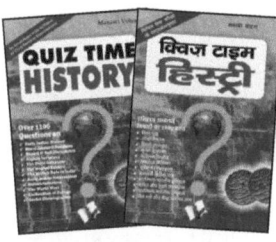 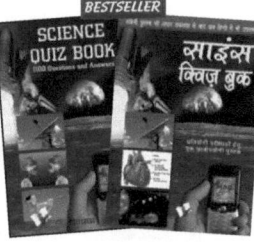 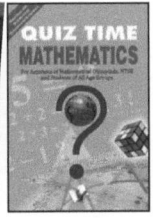 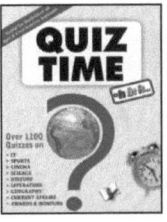 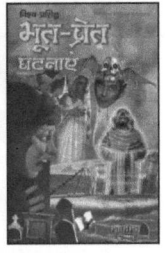 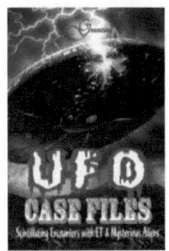

DRAWING BOOKS (ड्राइंग बुक्स)   BIOGRAPHIES (आत्म कथाएँ)

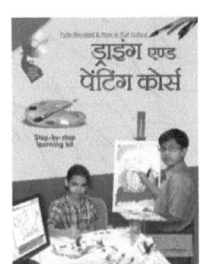 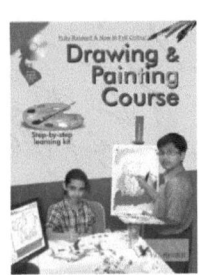 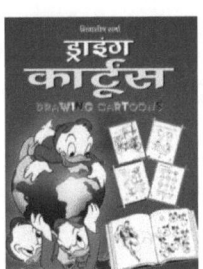 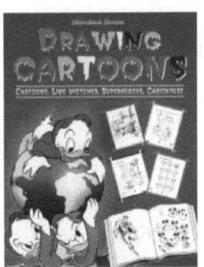 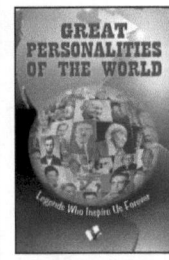 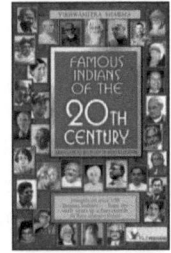

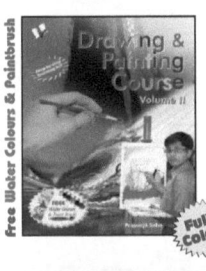 ## QUOTES/SAYINGS (उद्धरण/सूक्तियाँ)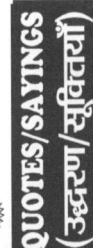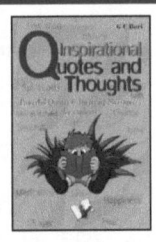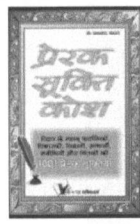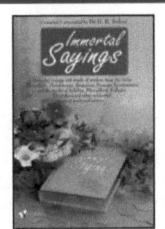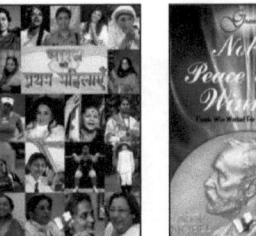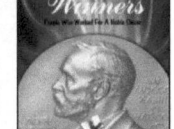

PUZZLES (पहेलियाँ)   ACTIVITIES BOOK (एक्टिविटीज बुक)

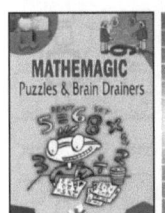 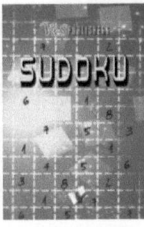 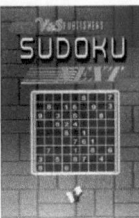 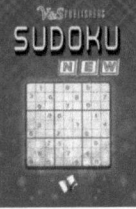 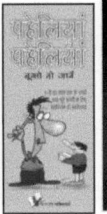 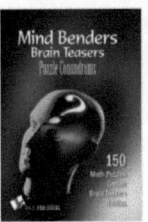 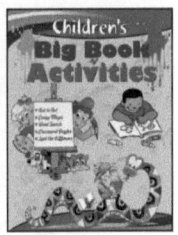 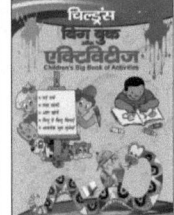

Contact us at sales@vspublishers.com

CHILDREN'S ENCYCLOPEDIA
(बच्चों के ज्ञानकोश)

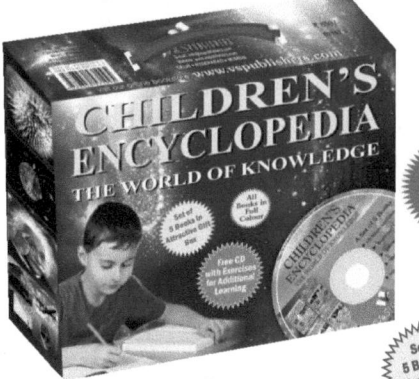
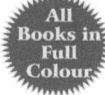
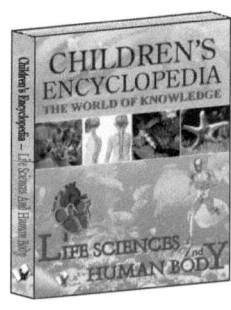
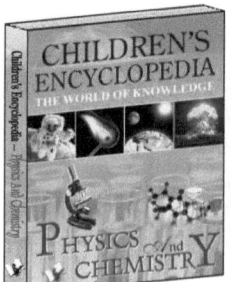
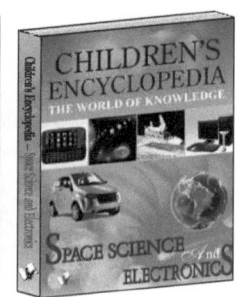
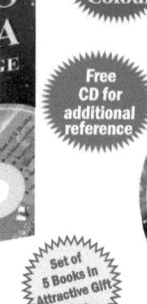
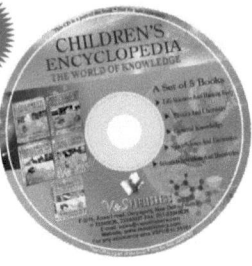
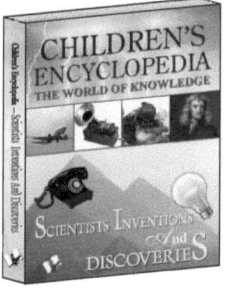
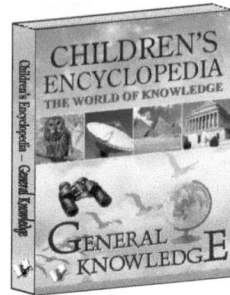

71 SERIES (71 श्रृंखला)

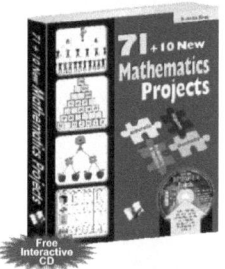
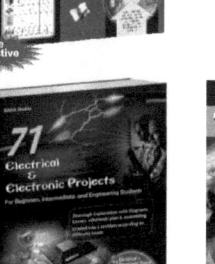
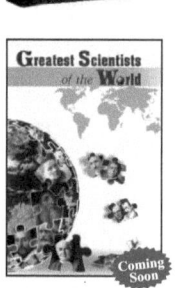
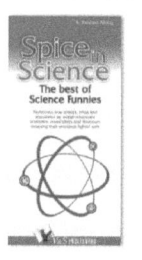
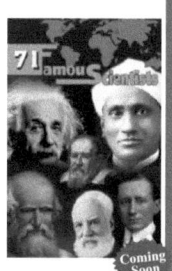
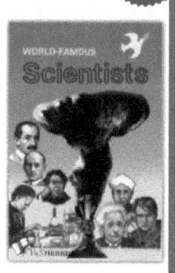
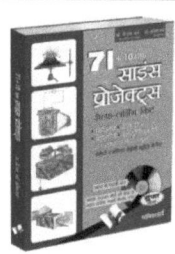
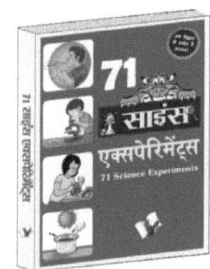
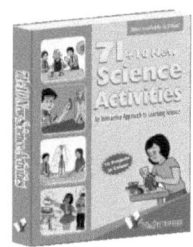
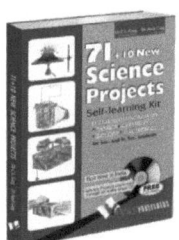
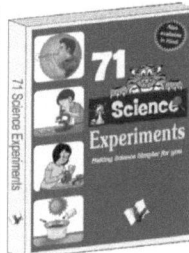
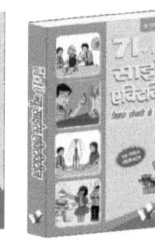
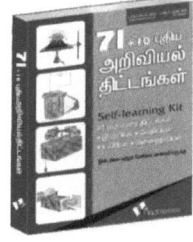
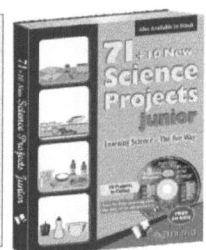
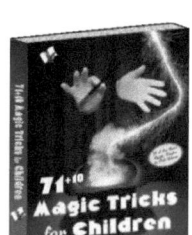
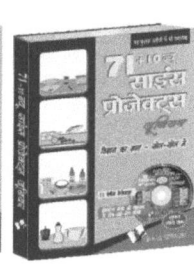
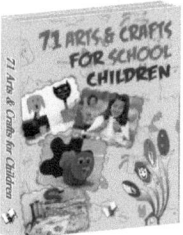

All books available at www.vspublishers.com

Printed by Libri Plureos GmbH in Hamburg, Germany